Good Habits

'A habit cannot be tossed out the window; it must be coaxed down the stairs a step at a time.'

MARK TWAIN

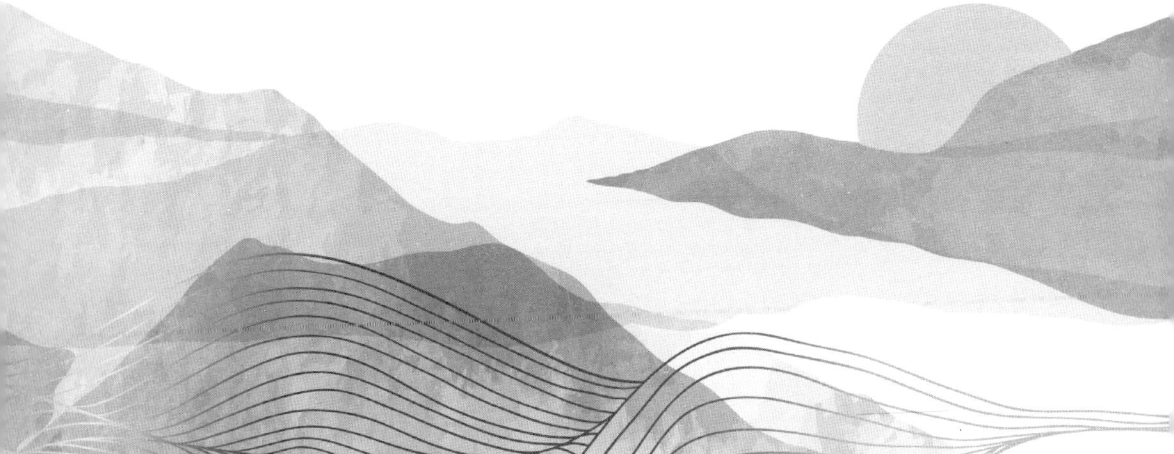

Good Habits

A GUIDED WORKBOOK FOR CREATING POSITIVE CHANGE IN YOUR LIFE

HERRON

What's inside?

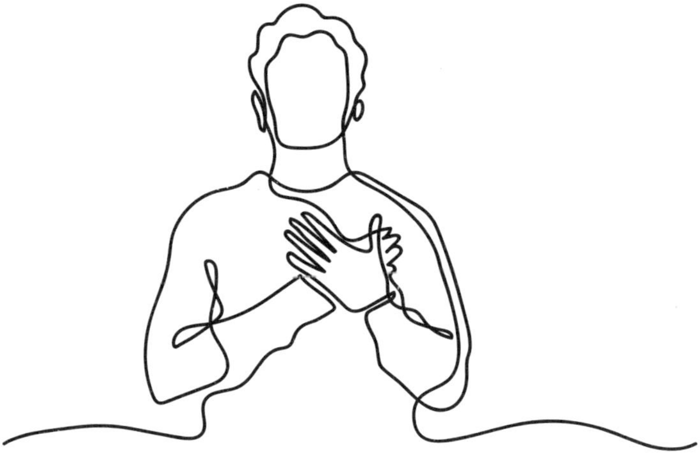

Introduction

Good habits are stepping stones to living the life you want and being the person you want to be. They are the building blocks of your lifelong project of self-improvement. How lucky: to be able to consciously build a better, happier life simply through awareness.

When we fully embrace this journey, we understand that the reward is intrinsic to the process, a process that is ongoing.

So set down your weapons, take a deep breath and let's get started.

Part One

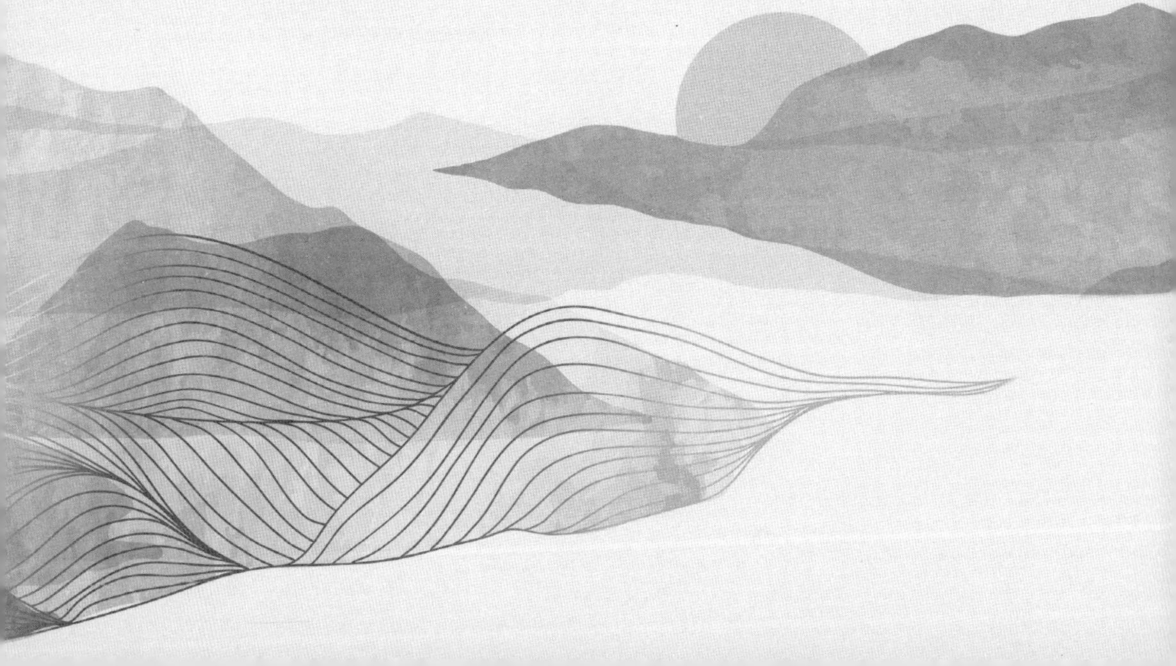

UNDERSTANDING HABITS

Maybe habits are not something you've given too much conscious thought to. What even is a habit, how do they come about, what is truly underlying your motivation to form a habit and, importantly, what are your habits, good and bad?

Answers to these questions, and more, can be found in the first section of this journal.

Turn the page to begin your journey.

It's all about you

Why does it matter whether or not you lose 5kg or meditate for 15 minutes every morning? If you think about it, the outcome is not what matters, which is a relief because chasing outcomes is hard. An outcome is generally a fixed and measurable event that signals the end of something. But good habits are here to stay.

So why do we bother? We might want to lose weight because it suits the mental picture we have of ourselves.

THE CHOICE TO CHANGE

In our minds, we are slightly fitter than in reality. Or perhaps we want to meditate because, although we recognise we are stressed, we know that within us there is the capacity for calm.

Without realising it, in our choice of habits we are searching for confirmation of our identity. It's empowering to realise this, because it provides a deeper level of motivation than an outcome can. Meditating is one thing, but connecting with the sense of calm within is a more fundamental reward.

You can demonstrate your commitment to yourself through small habitual changes. You can decide, 'I am a healthy person, therefore I take the stairs, choose a healthy snack, watch my portion sizes, do a few stretches in the morning, sit in the sun at lunchtime…' These small choices affirm your identity. It's not what you do, it's who you are.

Use the space provided to jot down why you want to change your habits.

What is a habit?

When we attempt a task, we usually: try, fail, adapt and try again. We repeat this pattern until we find the winning formula. Sometimes this is easy, sometimes it requires us to have a go, and then another, and then another. Eventually, the brain no longer requires the conscious process, and the task is automated. In this way, a habit is formed.

One of the big benefits of getting a good habit to the point of automation is that it frees up your mind to focus on new things. Habits, then, are not a drain, they are liberating.

Colour in the illustration opposite while reflecting on this affirmation.

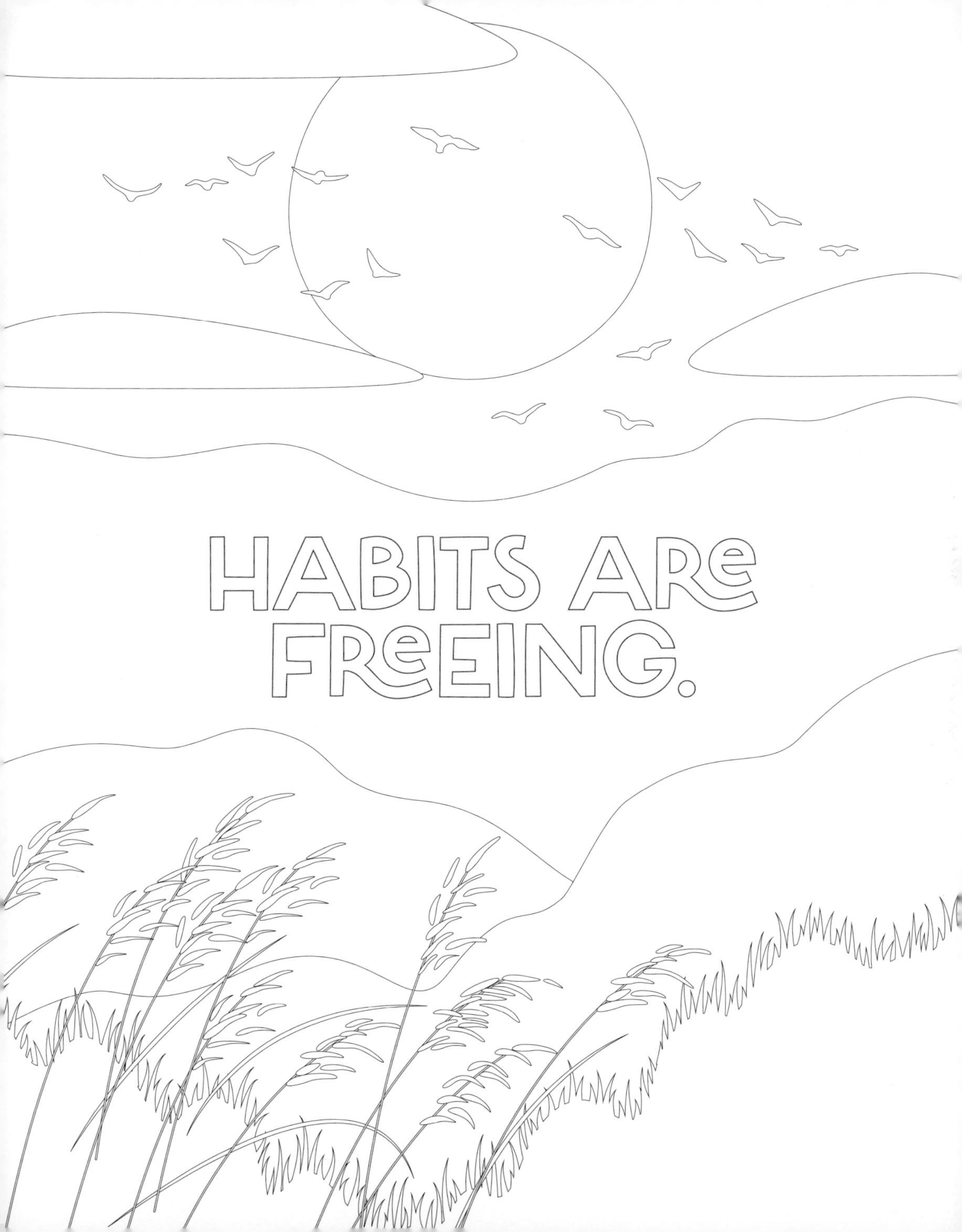
HABITS ARE
FREEING.

A habit is
a behaviour
that has been
repeated so many
times it becomes
automatic.

Loop the loop

In his book, *The Power of Habit*, author Charles Duhigg identifies a series of mental connections, or steps, that underpin habits. The Habit Loop is his term for this process of how habits persist.

The first step in the Habit Loop is the cue – the moment when the urge strikes. Next is the routine, or habit itself. And finally, there's the reward, which is the benefit you receive from doing the thing.

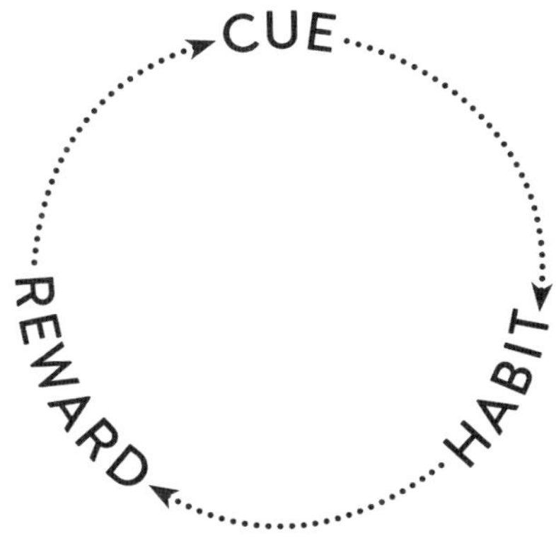

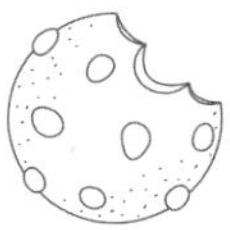

BREAKING THE HABIT LOOP

To take Duhigg's example, say you always like to have a cookie at 3pm – which includes a wander round the office and a chat with colleagues – and that's a habit you are trying to break. Here's what you'd do:

Identify the habit and describe it.
Pay attention to the place, time, emotional state, people and action that occurred before the urge strikes.

This is how Duhigg describes his 3pm cookie moment:

Where are you? *Sitting at my desk*

What time is it? 3:36 *pm*

What's your emotional state? *Bored*

Who else is around? *No one*

What action preceded the urge? *Answered an email*

What do you think is underlying Duhigg's desire to eat a cookie?

What's behind your habits?

Next, you get to play detective.

Use the exercise on the following pages to unpack one of your own less-than-desirable habits. Before filling it in, make a photocopy of this page so that you can use the formula to explore other habits in the future.

By completing this exercise, you'll get to review a 'bad' habit in detail, and hopefully gain a deeper understanding about your underlying motivations.

Once you know the motivation, make a plan to meet it. This is the easy and fun part. If the real craving was social interaction, you can drop the cookie but keep the same routine. At 3pm get up and find a friend to chat to for 10 minutes.

MY 3PM COOKIE MOMENT

What is the habit you are trying to break?

Your situation

Where are you?

What time is it?

What's your emotional state?

Who else is around?

What action preceded the urge?

Photocopy me first

CHANGING THE VARIABLES

Can you work out what's really motivating your 3pm cookie moment? Test out hypotheses. Swap the cookie for a chocolate bar or drink. How does that feel? Cut out the chat with colleagues. How does that feel? Carry on, recording the results of your experiment by immediately writing down three words to describe how you feel

I changed ______________________

I feel 1. ______________________

2. ______________________

3. ______________________

I changed ______________________

I feel 1. ______________________

2. ______________________

3. ______________________

I changed ______________________

I feel 1. ______________________

2. ______________________

3. ______________________

REFLECTIONS ON UNDERLYING MOTIVATION

By looking for patterns through this process, you can identify what it is that you are truly craving. What are your thoughts about this?

Habits brain dump

If you are looking to adopt better habits, you need to know your starting point. Bad habits (and some good ones if we are lucky) usually evolve without us noticing. It's only when we bring our awareness to the task of seeing our habits and actively trying to change them that we realise what it is we are really doing.

Before you begin the activities in this journal, here is your chance to take a tally of your current habits – good, bad and neutral.

To do this, first list all the habits you can think of. Go through your daily routine from the moment you get up to when your head hits the pillow.

Brushing or flossing your teeth is a habit. Tea or coffee? That's a habit. Where you hang your towel, where you sit to put on your shoes. Cereal on Wednesday and eggs on Thursday – habits. How often you check your phone, where you have lunch, exercise routines. You get the picture.

Your days are littered with habits, big and small, significant and inconsequential.

MY CURRENT HABITS

NOTE: *If you're having trouble thinking of all your habits refer to part 5, page 222 for some ideas.*

'And once you understand that habits can change, you have the freedom – and the responsibility – to remake them.'

CHARLES DUHIGG

Habits scorecard

Now that you've completed your habit brain dump, it's time to score your habits.

If you're unsure, remember that a good habit contributes towards you being the person you want to be. A bad habit might be enjoyable in the moment, but it's leading you down the wrong path.

If a habit is neutral, it's likely to be something you do that you can't attach any significance to – good or bad – even though you've thought about it. An example of that might be the choice of route to walk to the park, or how you file your paperwork.

HABITS SCORECARD

GOOD HABIT | BAD HABIT | NEUTRAL

HABITS SCORECARD

	GOOD HABIT	BAD HABIT	NEUTRAL
	♡	✗	▭
	♡	✗	▭
	♡	✗	▭
	♡	✗	▭
	♡	✗	▭
	♡	✗	▭
	♡	✗	▭
	♡	✗	▭

HABITS SCORECARD

	GOOD HABIT	BAD HABIT	NEUTRAL
	♡	✕	▭
	♡	✕	▭
	♡	✕	▭
	♡	✕	▭
	♡	✕	▭
	♡	✕	▭
	♡	✕	▭
	♡	✕	▭

HABITS SCORECARD

GOOD HABIT | BAD HABIT | NEUTRAL

Good, bad and neutral

When you have completed your scorecard, break down your good, bad and neutral habits into separate lists on the following pages.

You can add to your good habits list as you adopt new habits while working through this journal, and strike through bad habits as you successfully eliminate them.

MY GOOD HABITS

Write down your good habits – things you would definitely like to continue in the future. Ask yourself why these habits are good for you, and write down the answer here.

GOOD HABITS	WHY IS THIS GOOD FOR ME?

GOOD HABITS	WHY IS THIS GOOD FOR ME?

GOOD HABITS	WHY IS THIS GOOD FOR ME?

GOOD HABITS	WHY IS THIS GOOD FOR ME?

GOOD HABITS	WHY IS THIS GOOD FOR ME?

MY NEUTRAL HABITS

Write down your neutral habits. Ask yourself why do you these things, and make a note of the answer here. See if a habit can be moved to 'good' or 'bad' as a consequence.

NEUTRAL HABITS	WHY DO I DO THIS?

NEUTRAL HABITS	WHY DO I DO THIS?

NEUTRAL HABITS	WHY DO I DO THIS?

NEUTRAL HABITS	WHY DO I DO THIS?

MY BAD HABITS

Write down your bad habits. Consider what is wrong with this habit (why is it unhelpful for you), and make a note of the answer here.

BAD HABITS	WHAT IS WRONG WITH THIS?

BAD HABITS	WHAT IS WRONG WITH THIS?

BAD HABITS	WHAT IS WRONG WITH THIS?

BAD HABITS	WHAT IS WRONG WITH THIS?

Part Two

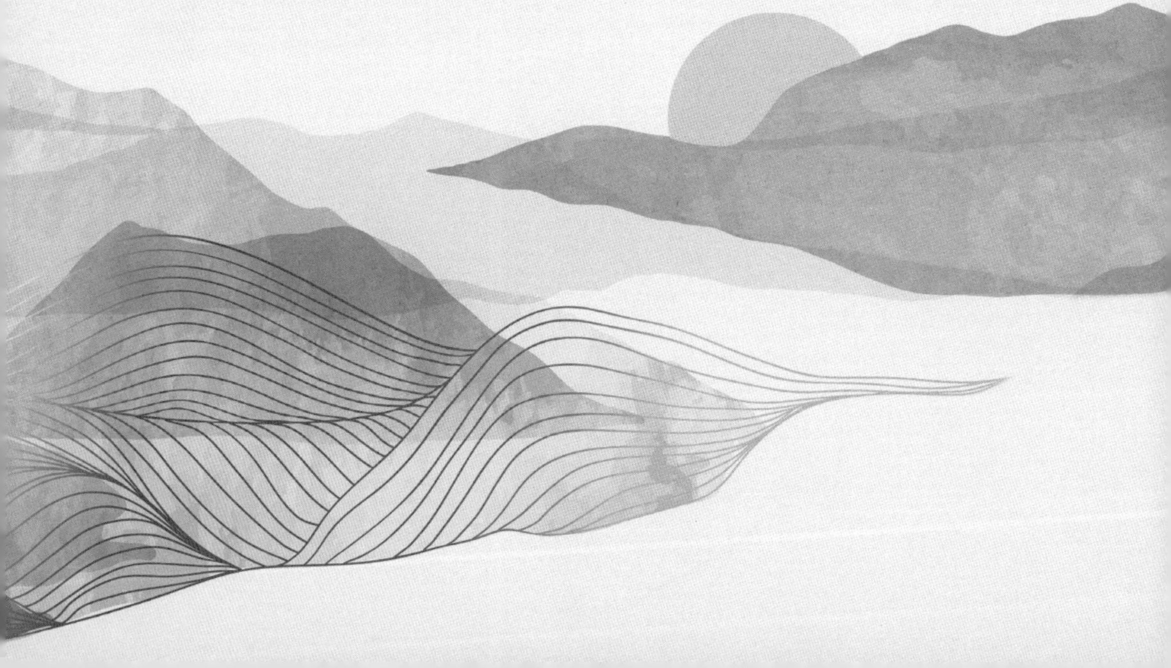

TECHNIQUES FOR GOOD HABITS

It's all about learning how to introduce more good habits into your life (and kicking the unhelpful ones to the kerb).

In this section of the journal, you'll learn fifteen practical and actionable techniques to help you do just that.

ONE

The Big Tiny

Tiny changes can have a disproportionately big impact.

In his groundbreaking book, *Atomic Habits*, author James Clear points out that if you put in 1% effort each day, you'll end up 37 times better over the course of a year. Clear refers to this principle when he explains, 'Habits are the compound interest of self-improvement'.

Little by little these tiny habits add up to huge improvements in the quality of your life, and ensure that you are putting yourself on the path to success.

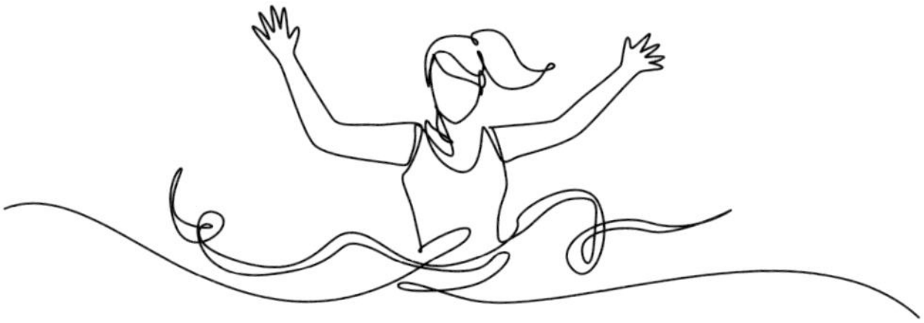

Patience. Keep going without obvious achievement. When you succeed, people will say it came from nowhere. Only you will know the effort it took. Success is the accumulation of small things repeated.

Winners and losers

Consider your life. Pretty much everything about it is the way it is because of your habits. That might sound like a radical statement but think about it: how you've chosen to manage money has played a big part in determining your wealth and financial security, whether or not you prioritise organisation dictates the levels of tidiness in your life, even your health, to some degree, is determined by your decisions.

Seemingly small, individual choices often determine the bigger outcomes of our life. When deciding which new habits to focus on, remember to put them in the context of your life and where you are heading. That way you can determine which changes will add up to a big improvement in your life over time – your '1% winners'.

The converse is also worth paying attention to. The '1% losers' are habits that you can let go and get a relatively greater benefit in return.

MY 1% WINNERS

In the left column, write down the habits you currently have that 'punch above their weight' – delivering a greater benefit than the effort you need to put in to do them. In the right column write down ideas for habits you could introduce that might have the 1% factor.

MY 1% LOSERS

Write down any small habits that you know are not helpful (do you need that second coffee? Think of the $$ you could save!) Refer back to this list later in the journal when you need a reminder of habits to lose.

— TWO

Jump on Board

If you want to start a new habit, but you are not sure where to begin, a good place is with an existing habit that you can use as a jumping off point. The idea is to link your desired behaviour with something you already do.

If you build a new habit into existing routines, you create an expanded set of routines that operate together – **think of it like catching a few good waves in a row, culminating in a great set.**

You can insert new habits anywhere into your current routine, for example: shower, brush teeth, change for bed, *grind coffee for the morning*, check windows and doors, go to bed.

Good habits
roll together

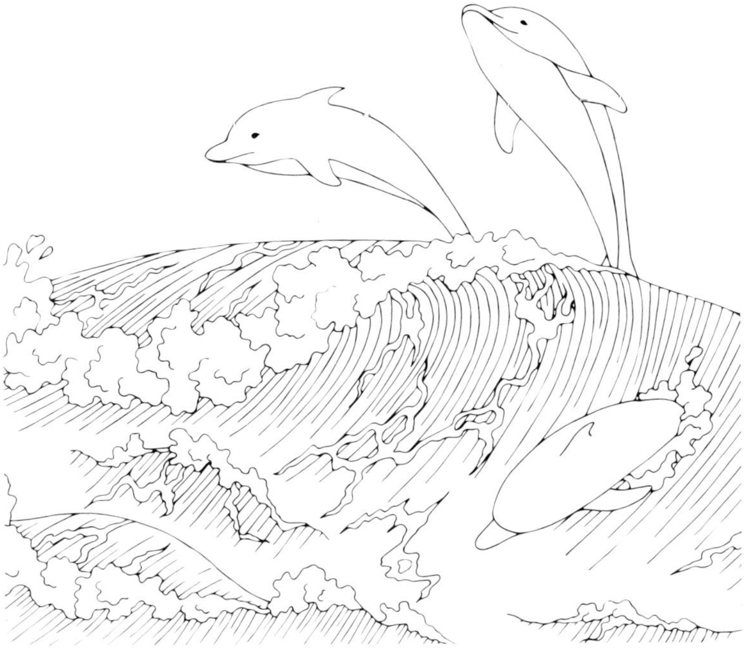

After: Existing habit

I will: New habit

Photocopy me first

— THREE

The Pleasure Principle

'Success is getting what you want. Happiness is wanting what you get.'

DALE CARNEGIE

Desire is noisy. It demands your attention and deserves your respect, because without it you probably wouldn't bother. Harness this potential motivation by using an understanding of desire – and its sidekick pleasure – to be successful in your habit-changing behaviour.

Desire and pleasure. The two are a little different. Pleasure is, well, pleasurable – we all enjoy the things we enjoy. But desire is about craving, and craving, as we know, is a catalyst for the action we know as habit. It is the anticipation of the reward that drives our commitment to the action.

So it's time to work out a way to make your new habits attractive. One way is to create a connection between something you have to do (the habit) with something you want to do (something you enjoy) and keep doing the two things in tandem until they become subconsciously linked.

Here are a couple of examples of how you can attach a new habit to something pleasurable:

While:

Drinking my morning coffee

I will:

Deal with my bills.

While:

Having a shower

I will:

Charge my phone.

Start small with these kinds of daily activities until you master the art. Complete the exercise on the next pages to get started.

Complete your list of pleasurable activities and target habits in the columns on this spread. Then create a line that might link any of the two activities, and move on to the next exercise.

PLEASURABLE ACTIVITIES	TARGET HABITS

PLEASURABLE ACTIVITIES

TARGET HABITS

Select four of your linked activities and habits from the previous page to begin experimenting, using the formula provided.

When I: (insert pleasurable activity)
I will: (insert target habit).

P.S. Cut them out and put them somewhere handy as reminders.

When I:

I will:

When I:

I will:

When I:

I will:

When I:

I will:

Photocopy me first

FOUR

See It, Do It

This is a simple one. We can make it easier (or harder) for ourselves to do something depending on whether or not it is visible.

Consider the water bottle on your desk. You are more likely to drink from it if it's there in front of you than you are to get up, go get a glass, go to the water filter and risk an unwanted interaction with a co-worker.

The inverse is true too. If you are trying not to check your phone as often, keep it in your bag or put it in another room. If the remote control is right there by the couch, there's more temptation to turn the TV on.

Think beyond your immediate surroundings for visual clues. If you want a different perspective, try walking a different route to work. Or if you want to eat more healthily, try shopping in a different store with more suitable options.

IN VIEW HABITS

Easy said. Easy done? It's never quite that simple somehow.
Get started by making a list of what you can do to put habits in view.

HABITS I WANT IN VIEW

HOW TO MAKE THEM VISIBLE

OUT OF VIEW HABITS

Then list what you can do to get habits out of view.

HABITS I WANT OUT OF VIEW

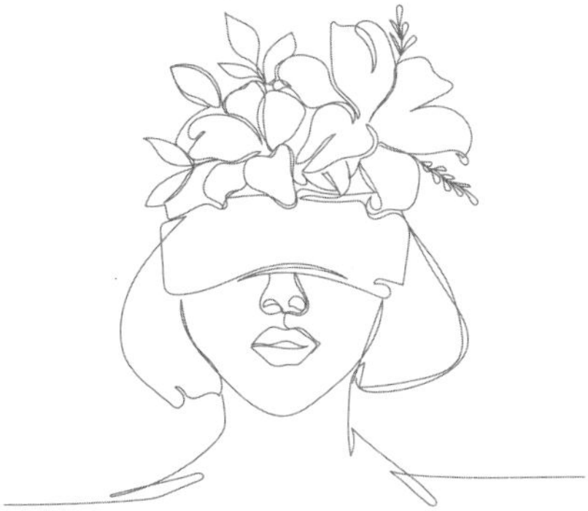

HOW TO MAKE THEM INVISIBLE

FIVE

Sing It

Sing if you like, but saying it will do. The point is to articulate and verbalise your intentions. To articulate means to state it clearly and unequivocally – and to be specific.

Take alcohol as an example. This is something a lot of people struggle with. If it is a habit you want to break, you could clearly state your intention not to drink alcohol anymore. Next time you are tempted to have a drink (whether or not you are offered one), say out loud 'I don't drink alcohol'.

Or, let's say you are a bit of a forgetful person and you want to address that. You really want to leave the house with all your things. As you close the door, be sure to state your intentions out loud, specifying the time and location: 'I'm leaving the house now, with my keys, wallet and phone'.

MY INTENTION STATEMENTS

Start by identifying one to six areas where you'd like to see change. These might be challenging issues (like quitting alcohol) or seemingly trivial, like dressing more smartly or eating less butter. Then write down your intention statements in the spaces provided. Remember to be as specific as possible.

Write it nice and big and decorate it if you wish.

E.g. I always look smart and presentable at work.

I don't eat butter on toast.

I make my bed every morning.

I exercise on Tuesday and Thursday mornings.

Intention statement:

Intention statement:

Photocopy me first

Intention statement:

Intention statement:

Intention statement:

Intention statement:

Photocopy me first

SIX

Join the Club

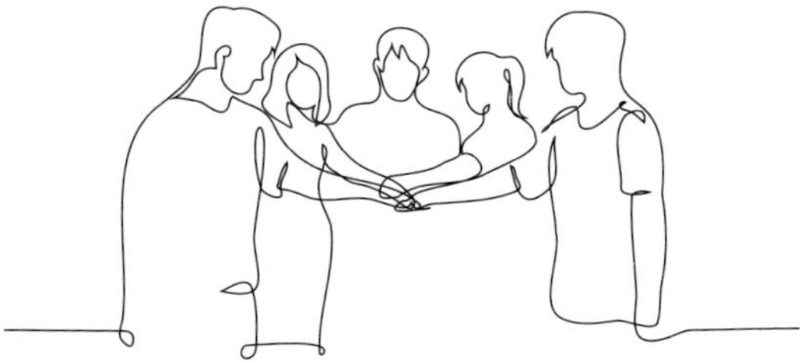

It's much easier to stick to things when we feel supported and respected; part of the team rather than an outsider. Surrounding yourself with like-minded people is a great way to initiate a habit, the basis of which is shared. You might sign up to bootcamp, and being part of the crew forms a great motivation to get out of bed and enjoy the endorphins with a side of socialising. Maybe you always mean to bake a cake for your child's school fundraiser but never get around to it – try joining the committee and suddenly it's so much easier to make a contribution.

Whatever your proposed new habit, think how it aligns to a tribe that you can be a part of and leverage those relationships and sense of community to make it happen.

PART OF THE TEAM

Complete the following pages to explore habits you'd like to adopt with the support of a community or group, and actions you can take to make them happen. There could be more than one group to approach so make sure to brainstorm all your options.

PROPOSED HABIT

TRIBE / TEAM

ACTIONS

PROPOSED HABIT

TRIBE / TEAM

ACTIONS

Photocopy me first

PROPOSED HABIT

TRIBE / TEAM

ACTIONS

PROPOSED HABIT

TRIBE / TEAM

ACTIONS

Photocopy me first

How are you?

Phew, you've worked hard to get to this point, but hopefully you're making great progress. Use this space for a chance to reflect and regroup.

SEVEN

Reframe Negative Thinking

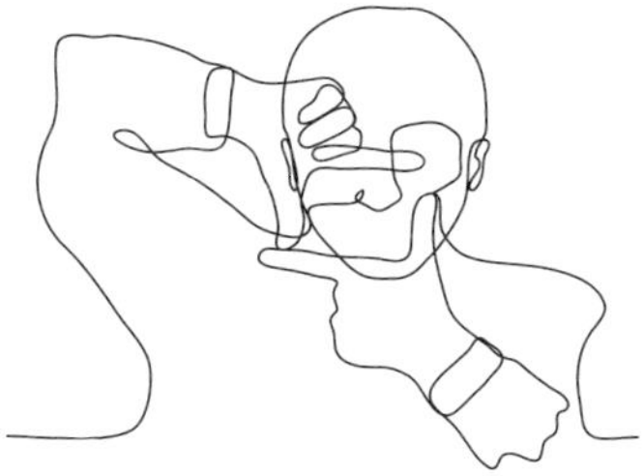

We often think of a new habit as a chore. Do I have to …? Let's face it: if it's not something that's naturally evolved for us, then it's likely to require a little effort. **What a privilege that you get to expend a little effort to make a big improvement in your life.**

Accentuate the positive as much as possible. Instead of thinking, 'Boring! I have to spend ages chopping all these veggies for the week', reframe it as, 'I get to prepare all these veggies now, so my life is easier all week'. Or think about how you can sell yourself on the benefits of exercise instead of worrying about the effort. Instead of, 'I have to get up at 6am to do Pilates', you can say, 'I get to start the day making a contribution to my goal of feeling stronger'.

CHANGING MY THINKING

How can you reframe a habit? List some habits and then select one to reframe. Once this has been successfully reframed in your mind, you can go back to the next habit on your list and keep going until you've done them all. Winning!

HABIT	OLD THINKING

NEW THINKING **REFRAMED**

HABIT	OLD THINKING

NEW THINKING	REFRAMED
	☐
	☐
	☐
	☐
	☐
	☐
	☐
	☐
	☐

HABIT	OLD THINKING

NEW THINKING **REFRAMED**

☐

☐

☐

☐

☐

☐

☐

☐

☐

EIGHT

Get Pumped

Create a ritual in which you give yourself a motivational incentive right before starting a new habit.

Over time this can reprogram the brain to associate the new habit with the positive feeling of the incentive.

It doesn't need to be an indulgent treat. It should be something that links to the upcoming challenging activity, perhaps a satisfying or calming activity such as a short meditation, listening to a favourite song or doing a few nice stretches.

My motivational incentives mood board

Brainstorm ideas for incentives here.
List them, doodle them or stick them in.

MY GET PUMPED MOTIVATION TRACKER

Pick one habit that you'd like to try and attach to a 'get pumped' ritual and track that habit over seven days, recording your experiences.

HABIT

GET PUMPED MOTIVATION

TRACKER		EXPERIENCE
DAY 1	☐	
DAY 2	☐	
DAY 3	☐	
DAY 4	☐	
DAY 5	☐	
DAY 6	☐	
DAY 7	☐	

Photocopy me first

GETTING IN THE MOOD

Music is a great way to create motivation and a common choice to help you feel pumped for a physical or otherwise challenging activity. The logic goes something like this:

Before going for a run I will listen to my favourite song. In time, listening to the song will prepare the mind and body for the run to come.

Brainstorm a list of songs that make you feel like getting into it, and use the list to create a 'Habit Pumping Playlist' on Spotify, or wherever you keep your music.

WHAT SONGS GET YOU PUMPED?

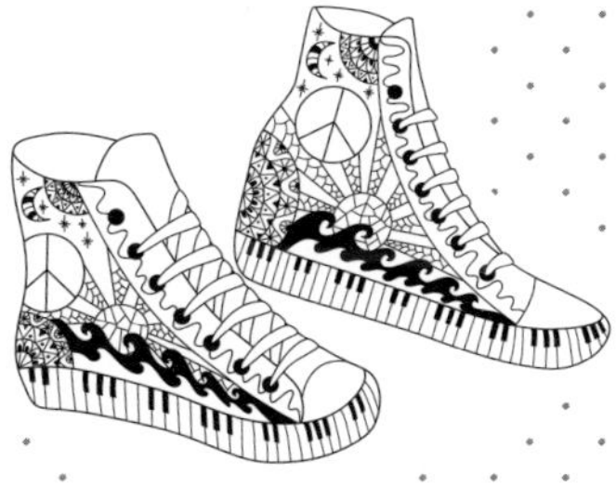

NINE

Do Something

Who doesn't love a bit of procrastination? We might not admit we love it, preferring to think of it as a vice over which we have no control, but the truth is procrastination has its appealing side that lures us in. It provides the opportunity to ponder options, evaluate pros and cons, make exciting plans, assess our skills, get lost in our dreams and thoughts – all the while delaying the potential for failure that comes with taking action.

But guess what: **taking action is the only way to begin and master a new habit.** Thinking about it won't make it happen.

CONSIDER THE FOLLOWING EXAMPLES ...

You want to eat more healthily.

So you find a few relevant websites, discuss it with a friend, maybe buy a book on a method that interests you, you even go to the grocery store and spend big on kale.

But until you eat that kale you are still planning, not acting.

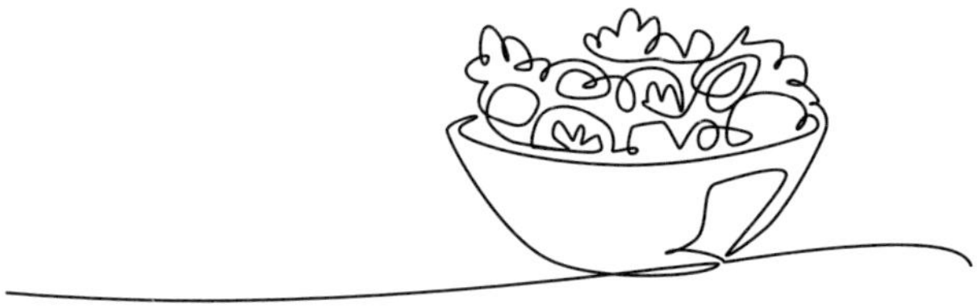

You want to start riding your bike to work.

You buy a new bike or polish up your old one, invest in some practical clothes and a backpack, get an app to plan your route, call a friend and see if they'd like to join in, you make a grand announcement on Facebook. You're all set!

If you had simply gotten on your bike and ridden to work, you could be a couple of weeks into a new habit by now.

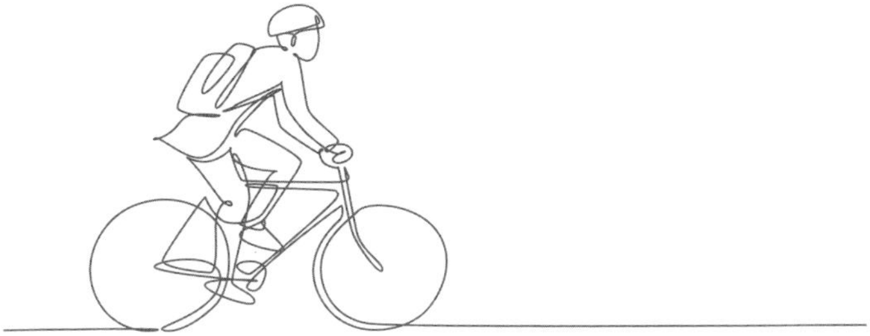

ACTION STATIONS

Use this space to reflect on how you can turn a desired habit from 'thinking and planning' (aka procrastinating) to ACTION.

1.

I WOULD LIKE TO:

2.

I NEED TO PLAN THESE ASPECTS BEFORE I GET STARTED:

3.

REFLECT BACK ON YOUR ANSWERS TO THE PREVIOUS QUESTION.

Are these genuine obstacles or procrastination?

GENUINE OBSTACLES	DISTRACTIONS
☐ ______	☐ ______
☐ ______	☐ ______
☐ ______	☐ ______
☐ ______	☐ ______
☐ ______	☐ ______
☐ ______	☐ ______
☐ ______	☐ ______
☐ ______	☐ ______

Photocopy me first

4.

IDENTIFY HOW AND WHEN YOU WILL GET STARTED ON YOUR NEW HABIT.

5.

RECORD YOUR PROGRESS.

Photocopy me first

I can escape my
thought bubble by
doing something.

Colour in the illustration opposite
while reflecting on this affirmation.

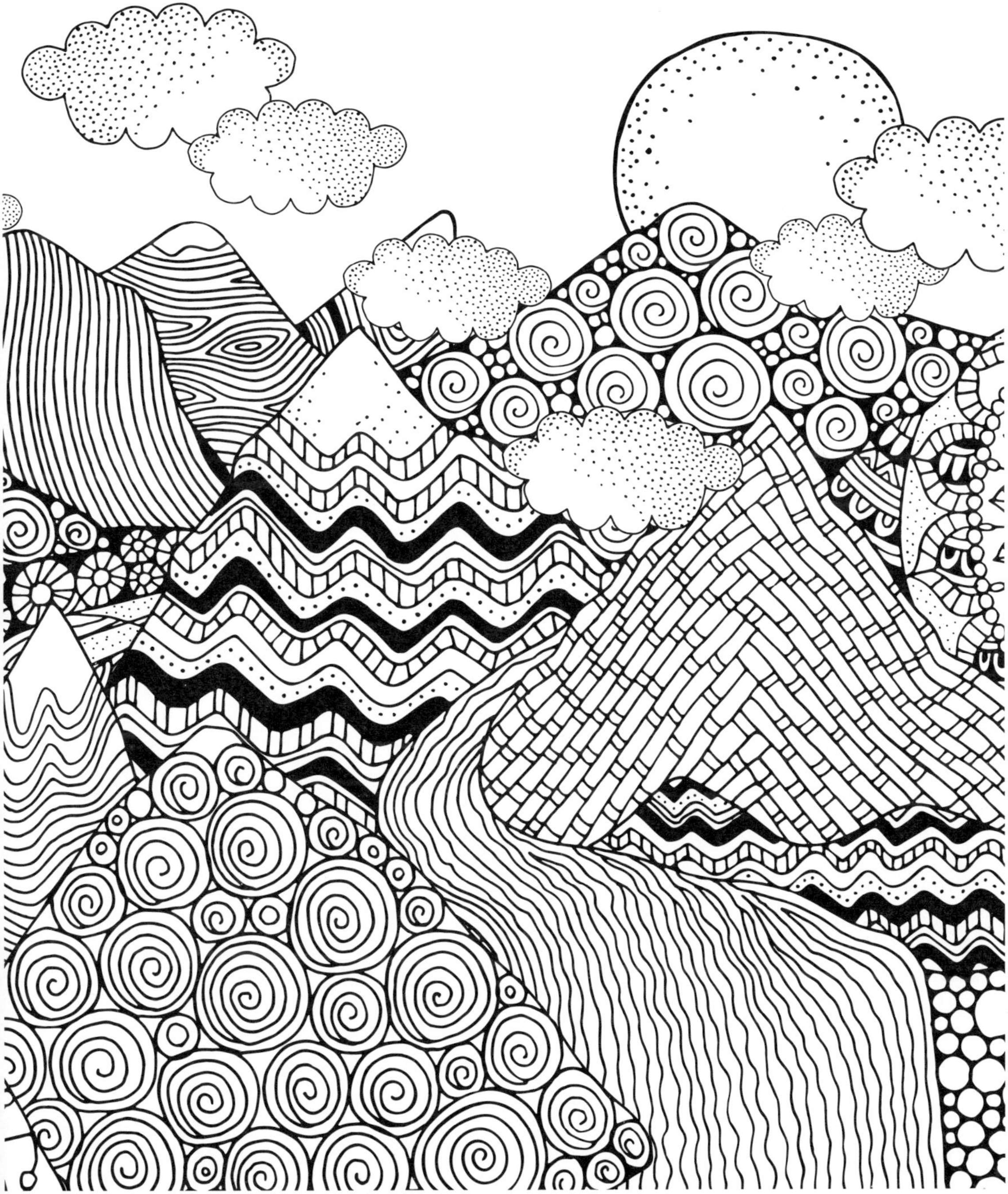

TEN

Practice Makes Better

Neurons that fire together, wire together.

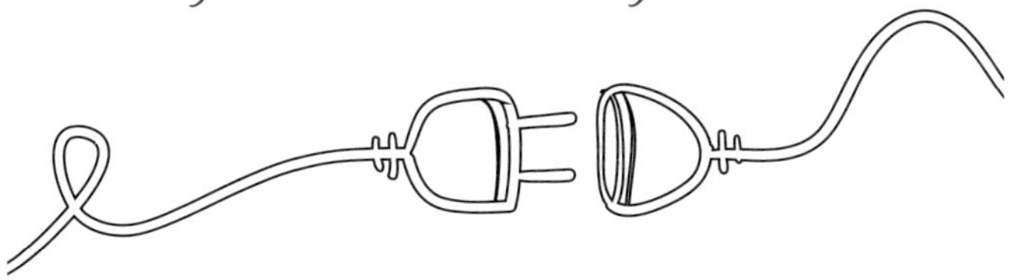

Neuropsychologist Donald O Hebb coined a phrase in 1949 that he'd probably be amazed to see doing the rounds as a social media meme in 2023, but that's what has happened to his words, 'Neurons that fire together, wire together'. By which he means that when you repeat an activity the structure of your brain changes to make that activity easier and more automatic. This can lead to physical changes in the brain.

If you want to master a habit, the first rule is to do it. Not once, but over and over again. In time, the brain will help you automate the process and it will feel easier and easier, up until the point where you barely notice that you are doing it.

MY TARGET LIST OF HABITS

Brainstorm ten habits (make them easy ones) that you aim to practise until they're automatic.

1.
2.
3.
4.
5.
6.
7.
8.
9.
10.

REFLECTION

What new habits can you fit into the existing flow of your life, and how?

How are you?

This habit business isn't easy. It takes work. Sometimes we feel like we are winning and other times it all feels just too hard. How is it going for you today? Shout, shout, let it all out in the space below.

ELEVEN

Make It Nice and Flowy

It's a fact of human nature that most of us choose the easy option. The harder the challenge, the more 'space' is created between you and getting there. To reduce that space, and make your habits more likely to stick, you need to make them easy to do – so easy, in fact, that you might as well bother. It's almost more trouble not to.

To achieve this, see if you can fit your new habits into the existing flow of your life, and create an environment in which doing them is as easy as pie.

Fitting into the flow

Habits that fit into the flow of your life are often things that make life easier. Getting cash out of the ATM when you will already be near an ATM at the same time each week, for example. Lock it in. Taking 30 minutes to exercise (a walk or a swim) when you take the kids to their exercise, rather than sitting and checking your phone. Good plan.

Here are some further examples of 'in the flow' habits you might like to consider. Colour in the ones that resonate, and use the blanks to add in your own ideas.

Make your bed! This is the ultimate example of preparing to make the next action easy.

Cut up veggies and put them in your lunchbox, rather than taking the raw ingredients to work.

Unstack the dishwasher at night and put lunchboxes out on the counter.

Set out exercise gear the night before.

Put tea or coffee utensils out before going to bed.

Recharge the Kindle before the battery dies.

When you run out of a grocery item, add it to a shopping list.

Prepare schoolbags the night before.

Return the remote control to its place when you've turned off the TV.

Place the watering can next to the hose.

MY NICE AND FLOWY HABITS

What new habits can you fit into the existing flow of your life, and how?

NEW HABIT

HOW TO FIT IT INTO THE FLOW

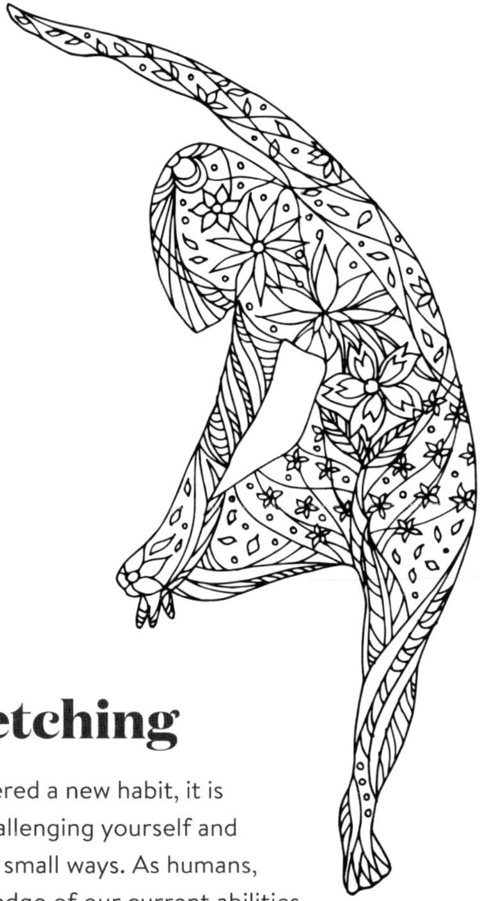

Keep stretching

When you have mastered a new habit, it is important to keep challenging yourself and continuing to grow in small ways. As humans, we work best on the edge of our current abilities. Too easy and it's boring. Too hard and it's, well, too hard. The sweet spot is somewhere in between, where we can keep growing.

'A mind that is stretched by a new experience can never go back to its old dimensions.'

OLIVER WENDELL HOLMES

TWELVE

Go Step-by-Step

The thought of new habits can be overwhelming. All the things to do and get right. Like most things in life, the first step is the most important. The detail of how things unfold after the first step is largely irrelevant because what will be will be. The rest just happens, but taking the first step requires you to make a decision and take action.

It might be a tiny action, like taking the herbal tea out of the cupboard rather than the coffee (after that you are 99% likely to have tea, not coffee) or putting your yoga clothes on when you get up in the morning (after that you are 99% committed to practising yoga).

What first steps can you commit to and increase your chance of having your habits happen?

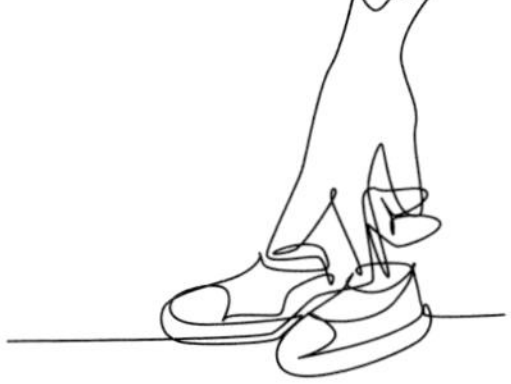

MY FIRST STEPS

Brainstorm five new habits (try to put some easy ones in the mix). Identify the first step you can take, and record your experiences doing this using the following pages.

1.

2.

3.

4.

5.

DESIRED HABIT

FIRST STEP

EXPERIENCE

I TRIED THIS

☐

I WILL CONTINUE

☐ YES

☐ NO

DESIRED HABIT

FIRST STEP

EXPERIENCE

I TRIED THIS

☐

I WILL CONTINUE

☐ YES

☐ NO

DESIRED HABIT

FIRST STEP

EXPERIENCE

I TRIED THIS

☐

I WILL CONTINUE

☐ YES

☐ NO

DESIRED HABIT

FIRST STEP

EXPERIENCE

I TRIED THIS

☐

I WILL CONTINUE

☐ YES

☐ NO

DESIRED HABIT

FIRST STEP

EXPERIENCE

I TRIED THIS

☐

I WILL CONTINUE

☐ YES

☐ NO

Then take more small steps...

Don't be overly ambitious when you want to commit to a new habit. Start small, so small you are maybe not even doing much at all, other than a glorified preparation ritual.

The power in this approach is that once you start it is easier to keep going – taking the next step is even hard to resist at times. See if you can discipline yourself to stick with the baby habit for a while, rather than rushing onto the next step. The idea is to show up for your new ritual.

You can think of this approach as a bridging strategy to get you over to the other side to an ongoing, productive new habit. You are getting started on your desired activity and proving to yourself that you are committed to your goal.

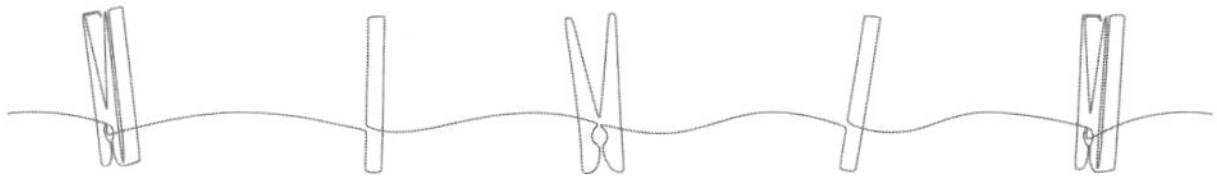

CONSIDER THESE EXAMPLES

Folding the Laundry

Instead of folding the washing before bed, you might commit to taking the laundry basket out to the table, or wherever you normally fold the washing. When you are ready, try folding a tea towel then leave it. Next time, fold a couple and so on until you find it's just easier to continue, and before you know it you have all the laundry folded and put away before bed (your ultimate goal).

Gardening for 30 Minutes a Day

Instead of jumping right in and gardening for 30 minutes on day one, instead get out your gardening gloves and tools and place them in the appropriate place. Next time, try weeding for five minutes. Over time you can build up to achieve your desired daily habit.

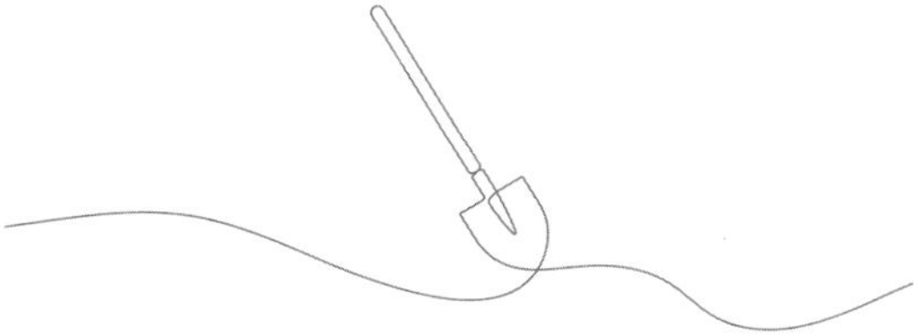

MY STEP-BY-STEP STRATEGY

Fill in the exercise on this spread, considering your long-term goal for your new habit and the smaller steps you might take to get there. Complete this over a seven-day period.

MY LONG-TERM HABIT GOAL IS:

MY BABY STEPS ARE:

1.

2.

3.

DAY 1	PRACTISED	
Step 1	☐ Yes	☐ No
Step 2	☐ Yes	☐ No
Step 3	☐ Yes	☐ No

DAY 2		
Step 1	☐ Yes	☐ No
Step 2	☐ Yes	☐ No
Step 3	☐ Yes	☐ No

DAY 3		
Step 1	☐ Yes	☐ No
Step 2	☐ Yes	☐ No
Step 3	☐ Yes	☐ No

DAY 4		
Step 1	☐ Yes	☐ No
Step 2	☐ Yes	☐ No
Step 3	☐ Yes	☐ No

DAY 5	PRACTISED	
Step 1	☐ Yes	☐ No
Step 2	☐ Yes	☐ No
Step 3	☐ Yes	☐ No

DAY 6		
Step 1	☐ Yes	☐ No
Step 2	☐ Yes	☐ No
Step 3	☐ Yes	☐ No

DAY 7		
Step 1	☐ Yes	☐ No
Step 2	☐ Yes	☐ No
Step 3	☐ Yes	☐ No

How are you?

Take some time to reflect on your progress and celebrate your successes, no matter how small they may seem. Keep up the great work!

THIRTEEN

Add a Little Sweetener

You might be familiar with the term 'delayed gratification'. It describes the process by which we act now for a reward that will come at some point in the future. It's a good habit to get into because 'future rewards' are generally more significant and impactful than immediate ones. But some people struggle with waiting and, for most of us, starting a new (and potentially difficult) habit can be made a little sweeter with an immediate reward.

Through reward, the brain ticks off on the new behaviour that it associates with pleasure. Over time, the immediate reward becomes less important as the benefits of the habit change become more obvious and intrinsically rewarding. For example, when you lose the weight you had aimed for, you no longer need a monetary or other reward for avoiding over-eating.

A technicality that's worth understanding is that 'bad habits' (like over-eating) often feel good in the moment, and bad only later. Whereas 'good habits' (like exercise) can feel challenging in the moment but good in the long term. So adding an immediate reward to a habit that delivers a positive benefit helps disrupt that process, and encourages you to stay on track.

ADDING PLEASURE TO GOOD HABITS

Use the space below to identify habits you can add a reward to – note both the immediate and the intrinsic reward (the longer-term goal you are seeking). Use the following pages to record your experiences and reflections on this exercise, or to add more habit-reward ideas.

HABIT	IMMEDIATE REWARD
Make coffee at home instead of buying	$1 into piggy bank
Don't look at Facebook	Make a social arrangement
Go to exercise class	Watch favourite TV show tonight
Try a new recipe	Icecream for dessert

INTRINSIC REWARD

Saving up for a new iPad

Do more IRL than virtual communication

Strengthen muscles and bones and improve mood

Improve cooking skills

REFLECTION

REFLECTION

I won't give up what I want most for what I want right now.

Colour in the illustration opposite while reflecting on this affirmation.

FOURTEEN

Look for a Good Fit

Habits that 'suit' you are destined for greater success. Sometimes we need to learn something completely new to achieve a goal, but most of the time we are choosing to focus on, refine and target areas of natural strength, or that deliver an outcome we highly value.

It all comes down to ability and motivation. Sure, you can do anything. But many things will be challenging, frustrating and time-consuming and you still might not do them very well. In other areas, you will make more rapid progress and the task may seem relatively easy.

WHAT MAKES YOU TICK?

In order to make a sound judgement we need to understand what makes us tick. Consider the following questions.

What's something you love to do but most other people might find difficult?

What comes naturally to you?

What puts you in the 'flow state' (where you are so absorbed by it that you lose track of time)?

What can you do more easily than another person, meaning you get a bigger bang for your buck in terms of effort?

What are your specific skills?

What do you really care about?

What is different about you compared to others in your social network?

What are some areas of weakness or things you avoid?

Reflect on any useful insights from the previous page regarding your 'good fit' and 'bad fit' habits, then use the space provided to list them out and note any ways you could do more or less of them.

MY GOOD FIT HABITS	HOW TO DO MORE

MY BAD FIT HABITS

HOW TO DO LESS

FIFTEEN

Embrace Boredom

As noted earlier, it's important to be both motivated and stretched in our habits. But there comes a point when we just need to keep on keeping on.

Regardless of a person's success in life, we all feel boredom at times. Repetition and practice are key to success in any endeavour. That's why it's frustrating when people give up so easily and, in family contexts, parents resort to comments like 'Practice makes perfect!' But it's true. At some point with any habit that delivers us a good result, we just need to keep going. It is boring, but it's worth it.

Stay focused on the result and the sense of accomplishment that comes from continuing to achieve in this aspect of your life.

Boredom blockers

Think about your 'why?' What is the reason you wanted to adopt a habit in the first place? Write your answers in the circles below. Refer back to this next time you feel the boredom blues getting in the way of your success. Hold them in your mind and press on. You got this!

How are you?

You've made it this far! Well done. Stick with us. Use this space for a bit of a brain dump and clear your energy for the next section.

Part Three

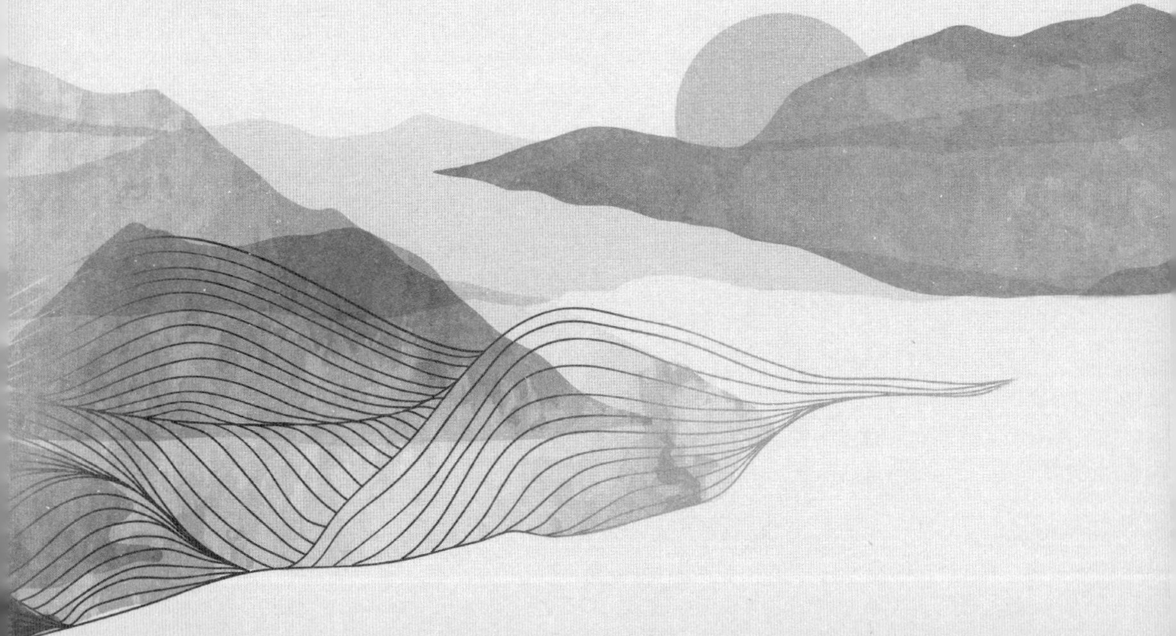

HOW'S IT GOING?

If you've made it this far, good on you. Hopefully you've managed to introduce some positive new habits into your life, refine old ones and get rid of those that weren't serving you very well.

Habits are work. And like all good work, they are better when we pause and take the time to reflect, learn from our experiences and reset the direction of our energy and focus.

Staying on track and getting a nudge in the right direction when you need it: that is what part three of the journal is designed to help you do.

Keep going

In order not to break the chain of your effort and momentum in pursuing a new habit, don't let one miss or oversight stop you from trying again. Remember two misses in a row is pretty much a new habit – and not one that you want! If you go off track, take corrective action. Scrolled your social media too much? Call a friend next time you grab your phone. Missed a workout? Get up early and do it first thing tomorrow. Splurged on impulse? Make your own lunch and coffee tomorrow.

One way to stay on track is to use a habit tracker. This is a simple device (see next page) that allows you to monitor your progress on your chosen habit. Evidence suggests that if you take note of your progress, your progress is likely to be better than if you don't. In addition, keeping track of your progress encourages honesty. It's harder to ignore when it's down in black and white.

Most importantly, a habit tracker is a motivational tool. Seeing ticks encourages us to keep going, and gives us a boost of satisfaction.

TIPS

Make it easy by using technology to automate your progress. Think fitbit or meditation app.

Stay connected to your purpose. Some of us have a tendency to chase numbers and ticks in tickboxes. That's good for motivation, but remember the bigger picture of what you are doing and why.

A CAVEAT

Some people see habit tracking as just another habit on top of a habit. It's not for everyone. If you are not the tracking type, just do instead.

Habit Tracker

Use these habit trackers to note your monthly progress. You can choose to track one habit at a time or multiple, and you can do this over one month or 12 (or somewhere in between).

HABIT

JANUARY

HABIT

Habit Tracker

HABIT

FEBRUARY

HABIT

Habit Tracker

HABIT

MARCH

HABIT

Habit Tracker

HABIT

APRIL

HABIT

Habit Tracker

HABIT

MAY

HABIT

Habit Tracker

HABIT

JUNE

HABIT

Habit Tracker

HABIT

JULY

HABIT

Habit Tracker

HABIT

AUGUST

HABIT

Habit Tracker

HABIT

SEPTEMBER

HABIT

Habit Tracker

HABIT

OCTOBER

HABIT

Habit Tracker

HABIT

NOVEMBER

HABIT

Habit Tracker

HABIT

DECEMBER

HABIT

Part Four

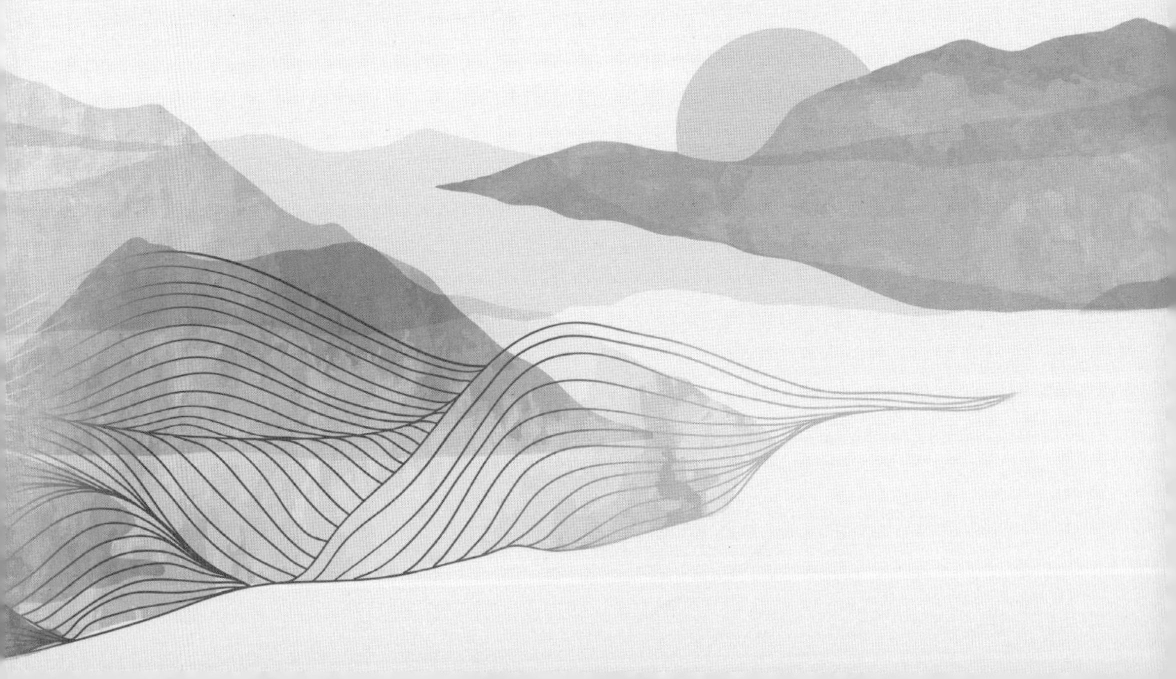

WHAT HAVE I LEARNED?

If you've worked through the ideas in this journal, the answer must surely be 'a lot!' Now is your chance to think about it and get a little more specific with your reflections.

On the following pages, you can review each activity set out in part two of this journal, providing your reflections on your experiences doing them.

1. The Big Tiny

2. Jump on Board

3. The Pleasure Principle

4. See It, Do It

5. Sing It

6. Join the Club

7. Reframe Negative Thinking

8. Get Pumped

9. Do *Something*

10. Practice Makes Better

11. Make It Nice and Flowy

12. Go Step-by-Step

13. Add a Little Sweetener

14. Look for a Good Fit

15. Embrace Boredom

'You steadily grow into becoming your best as you choose to be accountable and accept responsibility for improvement.'

STEVE SHALLENBERGER

Be your own whip cracker

If you are really committed to making a new habit stick, you'll need to hold yourself to account if it doesn't. Nobody else is likely to do this for you.

For example, if you want to get more sleep but you stay up late, what's a tangible consequence? You can create one. Perhaps it might be that if you stay up, you must donate X dollars to charity, or you will forgo television the next evening – or whatever it is that feels like the right sacrifice to you.

Decide on the habits that you want to nominate for that bit of extra help. These should be the habits that are really important to you, where you really want to see your changes stick.

DO THE CRIME, PAY THE FINE

Try writing your 'penalties' down. You might even like to have this signed and witnessed so that a significant other is helping to keep you on track too. See the example opposite.

Start with one habit and see how you go. First decide on your habit, intention, penalty and who you want to be your witness. Sign and date this document as though it's legally binding – but no outrageous fines needed!

We've created one for you on the next spread. Photocopy it a few times and keep one in regular view by sticking it on the wall or keeping it in your handbag (think of it a bit like that traffic cop trailing you on the highway).

PENALTY ENFORCEMENT NOTICE

HABIT

Regular exercise

STATEMENT OF INTENT

I will exercise on Tuesday and Thursday mornings

PENALTY

Friday pizza night is cancelled

PREPARED BY: Jen Dodds

SIGNED: J.K.Dodds

WITNESSED BY: Arkie Dodds

SIGNED: ADodds

DATE: 2 / 3 / 24

PENALTY ENFORCEMENT NOTICE

HABIT

STATEMENT OF INTENT

PENALTY

PREPARED BY:

SIGNED:

WITNESSED BY:

SIGNED:

DATE:

Photocopy me first

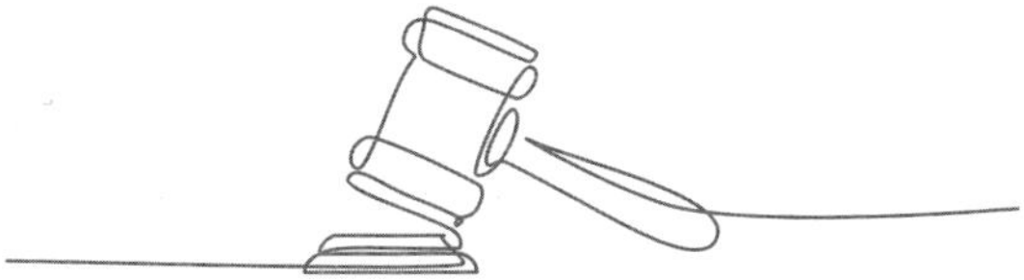

RECORD OF PENALTIES

Use this page to record any penalties you incurred for not sticking by your new habits. (Or leave it blank to give yourself a clean sheet.)

'Reflection is one of the most underused yet powerful tools for success.'

RICHARD CARLSON

Review, reflect, reset

Effective habits are fantastic – that's what this journal is all about. But if they have a downside it's that when we get to the point of habits being automatic, we can tend to become complacent. We forget to adapt and improve, or to consider how our mistakes can inform future habits. Every engine needs a little fine-tuning now and again.

FINE-TUNE YOUR HABITS

Do a regular review of your habits. Annually is a good idea, but you can do monthly or biannually – whatever works for you. Keep it simple and ask yourselves the following questions.

WHAT WENT WELL THIS YEAR?

WHAT WENT BADLY?

WHAT HAS CHANGED?

WHAT DID I LEARN?

HOW CAN I IMPROVE?

WHERE SHOULD I FOCUS?

WHAT IMPROVEMENTS CAN I INTRODUCE TO MY EXISTING HABITS?

WHAT NEW HABITS SHOULD I ADOPT?

Part Five

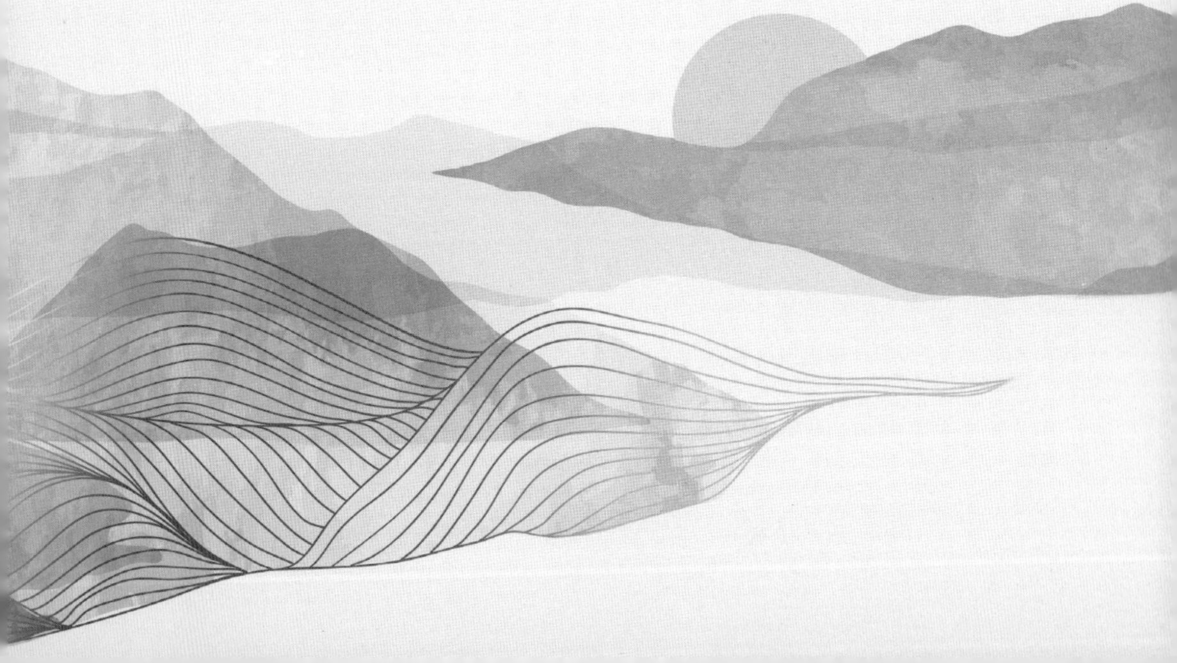

MINI DIRECTORY OF HABITS

It's not exhaustive by any means, but what follows is a list of ideas for positive habits that you could consider incorporating into your life. At times this journal requires you to think of new habits to use in an exercise. Sometimes that's hard!

This section of the journal is here to help. Have a look and see if there is a habit here that you would like to try out, or perhaps it will trigger you to think of another, better idea.

JOY

- Weekly pottery class
- Read daily
- Speak to Mum and Dad weekly
- Catch up with friends regularly
- See a movie regularly
- Go to a talk/watch a TED Talk
- Go to a concert
- Kayak monthly
- Weekend away every second month
- Plan school holidays
- Go for a bike ride
- Start a gratitude journal
- Smile
- Spend time in nature once a week
- Hug your friends, family and pets regularly
- Pursue a hobby
- Play a board game once a week
- Volunteer or help someone regularly
- Do a daily random act of kindness
- Listen to music
- Give compliments to those around you
- Join a dance class
- Enter a competition
- Try again at something you failed at as kid
- Send a card
- Do colouring in
- Be kind

WORK

- Use to-do lists
- Check email three times a day only
- Take lunch breaks
- Take a 10-minute break in the morning and afternoon
- Meet with manager regularly
- Wear smart clothes
- Always arrive on time

Never work on weekends

Network regularly

Focus on one task at a time

Do a two-minute walk for every hour you're sitting at work

Use time blocking to maximise your work day

Don't look at your socials

Be clear about your ambitions

Set career goals

Reflect honestly on your progress at work

SELF-CARE

Unsubscribe from ad emails

Try a social media detox for the day

Meditate daily

Quit smoking

Get at least eight hours sleep a night

Listen to a podcast

Read a psychology book

Learn something new

Create a daily mantra

Plan your day the night before

Avoid watching the news every day for a week

Spend some time outdoors

Spend time with positive people

Read, watch or listen to something inspiring each day, even if it's just an inspiring quote to reflect upon

Don't be so hard on yourself

Have a lie-down

Drink less alcohol

See your friends more

Make a new friend

Do something that's free

Help someone in need

Donate to charity

Have a clear-out

Pay for a spring clean at home

Have a facial or a massage

Eat out or have takeaway regularly

Have regular date nights

HOME AND FAMILY

Make the bed after breakfast

Unpack the dishwasher at night

Wipe and dry kitchen and bathroom surfaces at night

Clean the rangehood filters once a month

Wipe down the fridge interior once a month

Check use-by dates on pantry items

Regularly declutter your home

Meal plan once a week and try to stick to it

Eat dinner with the family

Stop everything and play or talk to each other

Regularly cook something new

Rearrange your displayed items

Put up the shelf, hang the pictures

Act quickly when things need fixing

Grow herbs and veggies

Do 10-minute bursts of gardening

Do micro-cleaning

Use beeswax wraps (not plastic)

Put the rubbish out (don't forget)

Put your clothes away immediately

Hang towels in the sun

Wash sheets and towels regularly

Minimise your wardrobe – less is more

Rotate your outfits

Organise your shoes

Deal with odd socks

No technology at the dinner table

No technology in the bedroom

Create an area of personal space in the home

Display flowers

Light scented candles or incense

Have regular family meetings

Give spontaneous gifts or cards

Say thank you to each other regularly

Share the cooking

Involve children in chores

Find something new and kind to say to each other regularly

Play games together

Look for conversation starters if needed (at dinner, for example)

Ensure storage is 80% full, never more

Nominate times for bigger jobs, such as gutter cleans, and schedule them

Schedule services such as pest control annually

Check in with each other

Spend time one-on-one

Keep outdoor furniture and other items clean and covered

Schedule car rego requirements before it runs out

Keep track of renewals for driver's licence, passports and other important documents

HEALTH

Set up regular medical visits

Schedule vaccinations

Walk daily

Stretch daily

Observe posture

Make time for exercise

Drink at least eight glasses of water a day

Try a new herbal tea each week

Eat fermented foods

Eat your five-a-day (veggies)

Eat the best food you can afford

Clean your teeth twice a day

Floss once a day

Drink a large glass of lemon water first thing in the morning, preferably room temperature or warm

Eat a healthy breakfast

Eat fish once a week

Apply sunscreen to your face every day

Get regular skin checks

Get regular mammograms

Aim for 10,000 steps each day

Eat one piece of fruit a day

Be mindful

Do a body scan

Take up Pilates

Try slow yoga

Go for a run

Join a team sport

Join an outdoor local community event, such as tree planting

Do a puzzle

Try two minutes of skipping daily

Stand on one leg for 30 seconds each day

Stretch your wrists after working on the keyboard

Set a timer to stretch every hour

MENTAL HEALTH

Meditate daily

Ocean swims weekly

Exercise three times weekly

Do yoga once a day

Begin and end the day with gratitude

Use a notebook to outline your daily tasks and goals

Stop procrastinating

Join a group – craft, reading, art, sport

Talk to others

Assume positive intent in others

Learn to set boundaries

Remove toxic people from your life

- Write and follow affirmations
- Journal in the morning
- Know and manage your triggers
- Record a line a day
- Actively quiet your inner voice
- Practise breathwork
- Pursue a spiritual practice
- Decide to be more open with others
- Practise speaking the truth, even when it is hard
- Create a morning routine
- Create a nighttime routine
- Practise good sleep hygiene

FINANCES

- Set finance goals
- Have a long-term financial plan
- Share finance goals with your partner
- Cancel Netflix or other streaming services for a month
- Call the bank to renegotiate your mortgage
- Monthly audits on ideas for saving money
- Connect with your advisor every three months
- Review payslips
- Review superannuation performance
- Review insurance premiums once a year
- Track your expenses daily
- Pay your bills on time
- Write down all your expenses and review them at least once a month
- Create a budget
- Use a shopping list
- Shop once a week only
- Make use of special offers or vouchers
- Wait 24 hours before making an online purchase that you had not pre-planned

'In a nutshell,
your health, wealth,
happiness, fitness, and
success depend on
your habits.'

JOANNA JAST

HERRON
First Published in 2024 by Herron Book Distributors Pty Ltd
14 Manton St
Morningside
QLD 4170
www.herronbooks.com

Captain Honey

Custom book production by Captain Honey Pty Ltd
12 Station Street
Bangalow
NSW 2479
www.captainhoney.com.au

Cataloguing-in-Publication. A catalogue record for this book is available from the National Library of Australia

ISBN: 978-1-922944-71-9

Printed and bound in China

5 4 3 2 1 24 25 26 27 28